Ebola Pandemic Survival LISTS

The 7 Lists that Show You How to Prepare And Keep Your Family Alive During a Pandemic Disaster

by

Jake S. Alive

While every precaution has been taken in the preparation of this book, the publisher assumes no responsibility for errors or omissions, or for damages resulting from the use of the information contained herein.

EBOLA PANDEMIC SURVIVAL LISTS: THE 7 LISTS THAT SHOW YOU HOW TO PREPARE AND KEEP YOUR FAMILY ALIVE DURING A PANDEMIC DISASTER

First edition. October 16, 2014.

Written by Jake S. Alive.

Thank you for buying *Ebola Pandemic Survival Lists*!
Want to save time checking items off your survival lists?
Visit my Amazon aStore at http://astore.amazon.com/jakesalive-20 to see some of the options you have for buying your pandemic emergency supplies.
Want to be first in line to get other critical survival LISTS?
The next book in the series is: **Zombie Apocalypse Survival Lists**. Get Jake S. Alive updates on free eBooks and other new books right in your inbox, by signing up here:
http://forms.aweber.com/form/31/2065881531.htm

DEDICATION

I dedicate this book to my niece Hayley. Rest in Peace, sweetheart.

ACKNOWLEDGEMENT

I would like to thank each and every preparedness organization in the U.S.A., and internationally, for making some of these lists available online. Granted, I wish they were all in one place, and this is the problem that my book solves.

ABOUT THE AUTHOR

The truth is I'm just a regular guy like anyone reading this book. I just went through the pain of losing someone to a COMPLETELY AVOIDABLE INFECTIOUS DISEASE before many of you ever did, and hopefully you never will experience what I went through.

I want to save a few hundred thousand of you from having the same heartache my family experienced when we had to watch my niece Hayley die of an avoidable illness. Make no mistake. *Unless you're in the health care or aviation fields,* **contracting Ebola is 100% avoidable if you act before the pack.**

INTRODUCTION

~ Knowledge and action lead to preparation. ~

Congratulations on buying the paperback version of this book. You are one step closer to surviving an Ebola pandemic emergency. Hello, my name is Jake S. Alive. I help people like you with families like yours to get prepared using these seven crucial lists, so you have a better chance of surviving a pandemic disaster.

By reading this concise book, you will have the seven lists that will show you how to prepare, so you can keep your family safe. And the key is you will have them in ONE place by purchasing this book. You just saved yourself numerous hours of searching over 22 emergency preparedness and survivalist websites to get this information. You're welcome.

I wrote this book because I lost a distant family member to an infectious disease. She was only 6 years old and had her whole life ahead of her. She didn't get a chance to grow up, make mistakes, fall in love, or start a family of her own. It was tragic and affected our entire family. **Her death was completely avoidable**, and if only we had the information you have in this book, she may still be here.

So I'm writing this book to save your life and your children's lives. No one needs to get ill or die needlessly when we already know that Ebola is on U.S. soil. Your best defense is knowledge, preparation and you need to start now.

Don't wait until there's chaos in the street, panic because of food shortages, and overall mayhem. Take some simple preparation steps now and give your loved ones a chance at a future after this first wave of Ebola.

SCOPE - What this Book Covers

~ Fear kills people. But preparation kills fear. ~
By the end of this short book, I want each of you to have gone through the list, check off what you have in your home right now, and decide which items you'll buy immediately.

I want you to know that I am not trying to scare you or fill you with fear. **Fear does not serve you or anyone during an emergency**. What I do want you to do is take these lists and do what you can to be prepared now. **Fear kills people. But preparation kills fear.**

One thing that all my friends know about me is that I was never born a survivalist. And I'm not a survivalist at all. But I believe in being prepared, doing the best you can to keep your family safe, and staying ahead of the chaos.

This book is intended for any individual or family who wants to **understand the essentials about Ebola and Pandemics,** and to have **the most crucial lists** of:

a) What to have ready in your home;

b) Items to have ready to take with you to an alternate location, in case you have to leave your home;

c) Items to put in your bug-out bag if you can't go to your alternate location by car.

This book is not intended to explain all the nuances of Ebola, causes, other pandemic emergencies, or suggest cures, etc.

You can find very thorough details on Ebola at the following links:

World Health Organization Ebola Virus Disease Fact Sheet – http://www.who.int/mediacentre/factsheets/fs103/en/

Center   for   Disease   Control   Ebola   Site –
http://www.cdc.gov/vhf/ebola/

Center   for   Disease   Control   Qs   and   As   on   Ebola –
http://www.cdc.gov/vhf/ebola/outbreaks/2014-west-
africa/qa.html

A   New   York   Times   Opinion   on   Ebola   -
http://www.nytimes.com/2014/09/12/opinion/what-were-
afraid-to-say-about-ebola.html?_r=0

Finally, I cannot dare to claim my lists are complete. No list is really complete because there are always options that work better for one family in one area of the world, while completely different options suit others. Don't lose site of the issue. The issue is do you have anything prepared? If so, check this list, and at minimum, it should get you thinking about your own preparedness for what is to come.

Ultimately, what I want you to do is read this book and start checking off the items you have. Next, you just need to decide what you will buy to be prepared before it's too late. This is your Ebola Pandemic disaster shopping / assembly list. For your convenience, I have intentionally left some blank space at various places throughout the book.

Read. Plan. Prepare. Be Ready.

A BRIEF OVERVIEW OF EBOLA

~ It will get worse before it gets better. ~

The World Health Organization (WHO) defines Ebola virus disease, formerly known as Ebola hemorrhagic fever, as a severe, often fatal illness in humans. According to WHO, the virus is transmitted to people from wild animals and then spreads in the human population through human-to-human transmission. The WHO statistic claims there is an average Ebola case fatality rate of around 50%. Case fatality rates have varied from 25% to 90% in past outbreaks.

The incubation period for Ebola is 2-21 days. Symptoms of Ebola include:

- sudden fever and chills
- headache, altered mental status (and even coma)
- intense weakness, muscle aches and pain
- coughs, sore throat and shortness of breath
- impaired kidney and liver function
- nausea, abdominal pain, diarrhea, and vomiting
- blood clotting is an advanced sign of the disease, and symptoms include:
- rashes
- red eyes
- bruises
- broken blood vessels in the skin
- collections of blood under the skin after injection
- bloody vomit
- spontaneous nosebleeds
- blood in bowel movements

- hemorrhaging (internal and external bleeding)

Note: Bodily secretions of Ebola victims – which incidentally are hemorrhaging out of every orifice! - are all highly contagious. It's a messy reality. Pun not intended. Transmission of Ebola has been confirmed through:

- blood
- emesis (vomit)
- feces and other body secretions
- saliva
- other bodily fluids, such as tears, or even sweat

Organ failure is the leading cause of death of Ebola victims.
There is no proven treatment or cure for Ebola. So WHO suggests early supportive care with rehydration, and treatment of symptoms to improves survival likelihood. At the moment there are a range of blood, immunological and drug therapies advancing to human trials. Thanks Canada.

In terms of the history of Ebola, the first outbreaks occurred in remote villages of Central Africa, near tropical rainforests. This 2014 outbreak in West Africa, however, has involved major urban centers as well as rural areas.

The Threat is Real.

And now it is here in the great U.S of A. As I'm writing this chapter, we are learning of the second health care professional who has been infected with Ebola in Dallas, Texas, who FLEW ON A PLANE from Cleveland the day before her illness was confirmed. The flight crew and pilots have just been put on leave to reduce the risk of exposure. Contact tracing is proving to be freaking crazy. It will get worse before it gets better.

WHO says that community engagement is the key to successfully controlling outbreaks. I say, start social distancing NOW. The key to mass outbreak control, in my view is not only "applying a package of interventions, namely case management, surveillance and contact tracing, a good laboratory service, safe burials and social mobilization". The keys are as follows:

- Arm yourself with the facts.
- Build your nutrition. Stay hydrated and healthy.
- Understand prevention controls (hand washing, NIOSH-95 masks, gloves, goggles – lists are next)
- Avoid Exposure (be ready to bug-in)
- Gather the essentials to protect your body.
- Set up a Quarantine Room (you may need one if one of your family members gets ill and you are bugging in.
- Prepare for when there is no doctor
- Review the lists below, stay positive and get ready to survive!

BEFORE YOU REVIEW THE LISTS

~ Preparation Pays Off. ~
For many of you, if you haven't watched shows like The Walking Dead or movies like Outbreak, you have absolutely no idea how bad things can get. I don't claim to be an expert, but what I will keep repeating is that preparation pays off. And once you knowing and completely understand what preparation helps you to avoid, you can appreciate the task, the costs and how you can save lives.

For this reason, I recommend that immediately after reading this book, that you find the following two movies and watch them. The more you know before disaster hits, the better a position you will be in.

RECOMMENDED MOVIES

Contagion (2011) - http://www.imdb.com/title/tt1598778/

This recent movie has been cited as a reasonably accurate preview of the pandemic scenario. Study it well.

The Road (2009) - http://www.imdb.com/title/tt0898367/

This movie gives you a realistic preview of the long term social and survival realities of a nuclear emergency, and complete shutdown of governments and civilization. This is the most undesirable ending for any family. Be prepared.

THE EBOLA PANDEMIC SURVIVAL LISTS

~Lists Make Life Easier. Lists can Save your Life. ~
The seven lists I feel needed to be included are:

1) BASIC PANDEMIC PREPARATION LIST
2) EBOLA PANDEMIC SUPPLIES LIST
3) GENERAL PANDEMIC SURVIVAL LIST
4) IN-HOME EMERGENCY SUPPLIES LIST
5) SANITATION AND OUTDOOR EMERGENCY SUPPLIES LIST
6) BUG OUT BAG LIST ESSENTIALS
7) BUG 'IN' PREPARATION LIST (FOR HOLD IN PLACE SITUATIONS)

Some important notes for you:

- You will find duplication in these lists. There are good reasons for this, two of which include:

a) If food shortages occur, or if law and order deteriorates, panic will ensue. *This combination of food shortages and increased crime should be your trigger to get out of major urban centers.* This is why you will want to have your bugout bag ready and packed long before that eventuality. So you can get out FAST.

b) A little duplication will allow you to have extras to stock up on. And if the emergency gets really bad or lasts longer than planned, you can use some of these extras to trade for things you may need.

- You may not know what everything on the list is for. All these items come with instructions and where possible, I've included some of the more important ones here. Once you buy an item you're not sure how to use, be sure to FOLLOW THE INSTRUCTIONS.

OK. Let's get to the lists. There is no time to waste.

LIST ONE: BASIC PANDEMIC PREPARATION LIST

¨ NIOSH mask (and consider an NBC-gas Mask, which covers you from Nuclear, Biological and Chemical warfare)
  ¨ Surface disinfectant
  ¨ Hand sanitizer
  ¨ Nitrile gloves + Chemical-resistant gloves (double gloving)
  ¨ Disposable thermometers.
  ¨ Tissues
  ¨ Isolation gowns, exam gloves buffount caps (hair covers) and foot covers
  ¨ N-95 masks and goggles
  ¨ Antiviral tissues
  ¨ Heavy duty sanitizers, such as Steramine tablets, and antibacterial wipes

LIST TWO: EBOLA PANDEMIC SUPPLIES LIST (ENHANCED)

- Pandemic Mask (NIOSH-95 respirator).
  - Gloves.
  - Tyvek suit.
  - Antiseptics (apply to skin).

Soaps, plus sanitizers and disinfectants (for surfaces, not skin)

  - Steramine Quaternary Sanitizing tablets (for your food handling surfaces).

  - Benefect Botanical Disinfectant (for other disinfecting other surfaces).

  - Simple Green d Pro-5. Simple Green d Pro-5.

- Probiotic Supplements.
- Duct tape and plastic drop cloths.
- Goggles.
- Thermometer (analog preferred over digital).
- Adult Diapers
- Emesis (vomit) Bags
-

Medicine

  - Elderberry Extract (Immune enhancing, strongly anti-viral qualities, a homeopathic solution for colds, all types of viral infection, and even chronic lung conditions. The help with anemia as well, are slightly laxative, and may be helpful for colds, constipation, fluid retention, colic, diarrhea, colds, coughs, nerve disorders, back pain and fever.

¨ Electrolytes (plenty of emergency drinks).
¨ Facial tissues.
¨ Bio-hazard bags.
¨ Cloth diapers and adult diapers.
¨ Vomit bags.
¨ Laundry detergent.
¨ Portable radio.
¨ Water filtration system.

The MOST Basic Pandemic kit. If the list above is overwhelming, you can start by getting the items in this basic list:

¨ NIOSH mask
¨ Surface disinfectant
¨ Hand sanitizer
¨ Nitrile gloves + Chemical resistant gloves
¨ Disposable thermometers.
¨ Tissues
¨ Garbage bags
¨ Diapers
¨ Vomit Bags

LIST THREE: GENERAL PANDEMIC SURVIVAL LIST

¨ 5 gallons of liquid bleach per person of the household to sanitize everything

¨ 4 boxes of exam gloves (different sizes for every member of the household)

¨ Quality N95 masks

¨ Antibacterial Soap (with Benzethonium Chloride) or Hand Wipes for meticulous hand washing

¨ 100′ roll of clear 4 mil plastic – for setting up an isolation room

¨ Duct tape (Duct Tape) – for setting up an isolation room

¨ HEPA filters – enough for whole house air filtration

¨ Several boxes of Borax – for provisional toilets

¨ 25 lbs. of lime per person – for provisional toilets

¨ 50 heavy duty black 3 MIL garbage bags per person – for provisional toilets and garbage

¨ 100 ordinary kitchen trash bags per person – for provisional toilets and garbage

¨ 25 lbs. of kitty litter per person – for sick people's body fluids clean up

¨ 100 rolls of toilet paper per person – for personal sanitation

¨ 20 rolls of paper towels per person

¨ Washboard and Clothesline – for washing clothes by hand

¨ Laundry soap – for washing clothes by hand

¨ Good dish soap like "Dawn" or other aggressive anti-grease formula

¨ Water filtration and purification devices

¨ Water collection, storage and carrying containers

¨ Water, water, and more water

¨ Food storage – for all members living in the household (3 months minimum)

If for any reason you are anywhere near infected people, and if you can't afford a full-body hazmat suit and respirator, you may want to get the following for minimal protection

¨ A Tyvek Disposable Coverall Suite might be a very good idea (several) – check sizes.

¨ Safety Goggles and/or a Face Shield will help protect the eyes (potential point of infection).

A SHORT NOTE ON FOOD

~ "Thy food shall be thy medicine" – Hippocrates, 460-370 BC

~

Healthy body, healthy mind. Eat well and keep your immune system healthy, and you'll need less medicine when bugging out during pandemic emergencies and other disasters.

LIST FOUR: IN-HOME EMERGENCY SUPPLIES LIST

¨ Water, one gallon of water per person per day for at least three days, for drinking and sanitation – and easy to carry.

¨ Food, at least a three-day supply of non-perishable food – i.e. canned food, energy bars and dried foods (remember to replace the food and water once a year)

¨ Battery-powered or hand crank radio and extra batteries

¨ Flashlight and extra batteries

¨ Whistle to signal for help

¨ Dust mask, to help filter contaminated air and plastic sheeting and duct tape to shelter-in-place

¨ Moist wipes, garbage bags and plastic ties for personal sanitation

¨ Wrench or pliers to turn off utilities

¨ Manual can opener for food (if kit contains canned food)

¨ Local maps

¨ Pocket knife

¨ Machete for protection and travelling through any wooded areas

¨ Extra batteries

¨ Fully-stocked first aid kit

¨ Special needs items

¨ Prescription medications, infant formula or equipment for people with disabilities

¨ Extra keys for your car and house

¨ Cash

¨ Include smaller bills, such as $10 bills and change for the odd payphones

¨ Valuable items to trade e.g. Lighters, small knives,

¨ Additional Items to Consider Adding to an Emergency Supply Kit:

¨ Extra prescription medications

¨ Reading glasses

¨ Infant formula and diapers

¨ Pet food and extra water for your pet

¨ Important family documents such as copies of insurance policies

¨ Identification and bank account records in a waterproof, portable container

¨ Emergency reference material such as a first aid book

¨ Sleeping bag or warm blanket for each person. Consider additional bedding if you live in a cold-weather climate.

¨ Complete change of clothing for each member of your family or group, including a long sleeved shirt, long pants and sturdy shoes. Consider additional clothing if you live in a cold-weather climate.

¨ Household chlorine bleach and medicine dropper – When diluted nine parts water to one part bleach, bleach can be used as a disinfectant. Or in an emergency, you can use it to treat water by using 16 drops of regular household liquid bleach per gallon of water. Do not use scented, color safe or bleaches with added cleaners.

¨ Fire Extinguisher

¨ Matches in a waterproof container

¨ Feminine supplies and personal hygiene items

¨ Mess kits, paper cups, plates and plastic utensils, paper towels

¨ Paper and pencil

¨ Books, games, puzzles or other activities for children

LIST FIVE: SANITATION AND OUTDOOR EMERGENCY SUPPLIES LIST

¨ Shovels to dig an outhouse
    ¨ Buckets
    ¨ Heavy plastic garbage bag for emergency storage of fecal matter
    ¨ Disinfectants
    ¨ Bleach
    ¨ Toilet paper
    ¨ Washcloths
    ¨ Towels
    ¨ Feminine sanitary products
    ¨ Hand Sanitizer
    ¨ Moist towels / moist wipes
    ¨ Toilet Paper
    ¨ Soap / body wash
    ¨ Shampoo / Conditioner
    ¨ Toothbrushes, toothpaste
    ¨ Razors
    ¨ Shaving creams
    ¨ Mirror
    ¨ Comb / brush
    ¨ Lip balm
    ¨ Sunscreen
    ¨ Lotion
    ¨ Vaseline

LIST SIX: BUG OUT BAG LIST

Some explanations are provided here for your information and understanding.

"Bugging Out" is the decision to temporarily (or permanently) say bye-bye and leave your home behind, to get to a safer destination in the event of a large-scale disaster.

When you bug out, you may or may not be able to leave with your vehicle. This is why most preppers suggest you have a bugout bag stocked and ready to walk to your safer destination if needs be. Some preppers are really prepared on this one. They know what their 'safer destination' is, and they have a plan and a route to get there on foot. And guess what else? Some of them bury a separate bug out bag at intervals along their route to that 'safer destination'. Why? Well, let's say your safer destination is 5 days walk away from your home. 5 days' worth of food, supplies and essentials can weigh a LOT. So preppers bury bugout bags at 2 to 3-days walking intervals.

Look, I'm not suggesting you do that. If you do, that's great. But at least have one bugout bag per family member, all ready to go, and stored as close as possible to your front or back door for immediate exit if needed.

Here are the lists of items needed for a well-stocked bugout bag, sorted by supply type.

WATER AND HYDRATION

Most important, as the body can't go over 72 hours without water, yet it can go up to 3 weeks without food. Have a 1 liter minimum, per day, per person. Highly recommended. Here are the items that man sites recommend.

¨ Drinking Water (3 Liters)

․ Water Filters / Purification Systems
․ Water Purification Tablets (Qty 3)
․ Collapsible Water Bottle
․ Hard Water Bottle
․ Metal Water Bottle / Canteen

FOOD AND FOOD PREPARATION

Have a variety of off-the-shelf, dehydrated, store-bought items. Consider non-perishable food items, where some require water and some that don't, as there's no way to predict how scarce the water supply will be. Assume it will be scarcer than you think. Plan for enough food to last a minimum of three days. Also, take metal cooking utensils and cookware. They last longer and can't get busted on while you're bugging out.

․ P-38 Can Opener
․ Metal Cooking Pot
․ Metal Cup
․ Pot Scrubber
․ Portable Stove
․ Protein / Energy Bars (Qty 6 per person)
․ MREs / Dehydrated Meals (Qty 3 per person)
․ Spork (all-in-one spoon plus fork)
․ Stove Fuel (Qty 8 Tablets)

CLOTHING

Choose comfortable, warm, stretchy and breathable clothes. Pack in layers. Consider time of year and climate. You need at least two changes of clothes per family member (and 4 for children). That way you'll always have a dry set to wear and can avoid hypothermia.

․ Lightweight Long Sleeve Shirt
․ Convertible (Zip-Off) Pants
․ Underwear
․ Wool Hiking Socks (Qty 3 pair)
․ Medium Weight Fleece
․ Hat w/ Flex Brim

¨ Working Gloves
¨ Rain Poncho
¨ Shemagh

OUTDOOR SHELTER AND BEDDING

Don't skimp on these. Many come in lightweight formats and all of them will help you to be more comfortable in the elements. During an emergency that requires bugging out, you need a restful sleep more than any other time in your life.

¨ Tarp
¨ Tent
¨ Sleeping Bag
¨ Ground Pad
¨ Wool Blanket

HEAT SOURCE

Staying warm when bugging out can keep you alive and keep you eating healthy foods. The survivalist mantra around items that provide heat, light and protection is this:

"Where there are two, there's one. Where there's one, there's none."

This means you are a sure goner if you're primary item fails and you have no backup. This is why many recommend 3 or even 4 of the following items in your bugout bag.

¨ Ignition Source (Qty 3)
¨ Tinder (Qty 3)
¨ Waterproof Storage

FIRST AID

There are so many first aid kits out there, yet we know that some things in the kit always run out and others are underused. This is why you want to have some of the following additional first aid items ready.

¨ First Aid Kit
¨ Insect Repellant
¨ Mylar Survival Blanket
¨ Burn kit

¨ Extra plastic and fabric bandages

HYGIENE

Never underestimate good hygiene. Don't believe for a moment that you can run away from a pandemic, and that just because you bugged out, you're safe. There are worse illnesses you can easily get from improper hand washing and poor hygiene. These can be the little things that make a big difference when you bug out.

¨ Wet Napkins
¨ Hand Sanitizer
¨ All-Purpose Camp Soap
¨ Hygiene/Signal Mirror
¨ Small Pack Towel
¨ Travel Toilet Paper (Qty 2)
¨ Feminine Products
¨ Face tissues

TOOLS

Stick to the basics in this area. Not everyone can or wants to carry guns and rifles, so choose to your preference. And have 2 or 3 backups.

¨ Survival Knife
¨ Multi-Tool
¨ Switch Blade
¨ Box cutter
¨ Six to Eight Inch Serrated Blade
¨ Machete

LIGHTING and ILLUMINATION

Whichever you pick from the list below, have 2 or three backups. And remember extra batteries.

¨ LED Headlamp
¨ Mini LED Keychain
¨ Light Glow stick
¨ Mini LED Light
¨ Emergency Flare Gun
¨ Candles

¨ Batteries

COMMUNICATIONS

There's fierce debate on if and how much communication you should have when bugging out. My advice is: Have something. And a backup. If things go back to normal, you'll want to know!

¨ Cell Phone
¨ Crank Power Charger
¨ Emergency Radio with Hand Crank

TRAVEL AIDS

These are some of the items that can help you get from A to B when you're bugging out. Use them, trade them, and don't leave home without them.

¨ $500 Minimum in Small Bills
¨ Quarters (Qty 8)
¨ Gold / Silver Bullion Coins
¨ Local Area Map
¨ Compass
¨ GPS (and batteries)
¨ Small Note Pad / Pencil
¨ Emergency Whistle(1 per person in your group)

SELF DEFENSE / FAMILY PROTECTION

Bugging out can become a life or death situation. Not everyone will be as prepared as you. And in the worst cases of chaos and government collapse, the things you have can become highly desirable to someone who hasn't prepared. Carry some of these, and **BE READY TO USE THEM** to protect your family.

¨ Pepper Spray
¨ Bear Spray
¨ Long knife or machete
¨ Handgun
¨ Takedown rifle
¨ Ammunition (Qty 50 rounds minimum)

MISCELLANEOUS ESSENTIALS

Don't think you're out of the woods yet. Some of the things below can be of massive utility when bugging out.

- 550 Parachute Cord (50′)
- Cotton Bandana
- Duct Tape (25')
- 55 Gal. Contractor Garbage Bag (Qty 2)
- Re-sealable Bags (Qty 5, Various Sizes)
- Sunglasses
- Wide brim hat
- N95 Face Mask
- Sewing Kit
- Latex Tubing (3')
- Fishing Kit
- Condoms (Non-lubricated)
- Binoculars (Optional)
- Face Paint
- Military Surplus Survival / Snare Wire

LIST SEVEN: BUGGING IN ESSENTIALS

'Bugging in' is a scenario where you and your family decide to hold in place at home. Here's what we mean. There are times when bugging out is not needed or not the ideal next step. And there may be situations where it's impossible to leave your home. Bugging in is more commonly referred to as hunkering down. But again, as many people will not have prepared as you will have, a large-scale disaster can create additional health and safety issues for you and your family to deal with.

Imagine the following as a worst case scenario, and when bugging in is the only option:

- loss of power and water
- shutdown of local hospitals
- no transportation
- no city trash removal
- cut natural gas lines
- no phone lines of cell phone towers
- no grocery supplies
- no emergency services providers.

It becomes critical to prepare and to protect your family and your belongings.

The key to preparation is to consider stocking up for a minimum of two weeks (over and above your usual home supplies). Start there, and ideally, work your way up so you can survive for two to six months on the following bugging in items:

- Shelter
- Water

- Fire
- Food
- First aid
- Self-defense

SHELTER

Includes cover and heat during cold months. Some cost-effective heating solutions you can have in place are:

" Wood burning fireplaces
" Kerosene heaters
" Portable propane heaters
" Portable emergency propane heaters (for small spaces)
" Rooms identified to be closed off from heat
" Blankets (also to reduce heat loss at windows)
" Sleeping bags
" Candles
" Fuel for each heat source you choose.

WATER

Assume you'll have no water supply in your home. You'll need water for drinking, cooking, basic sewage, and for good hygiene. You can buy water by the gallon or treat the tap water in your home with a bleach solution (4 drops unscented bleach to 1 gallon of water) and store them in empty gallon containers or sanitized 2L bottles (sanitize using a solution of 1tsp bleach to 1 quart water). Things you'll need:

" A few gallons of unscented household bleach (to purify water and for other sanitation needs)
" Containers to collect water (even your bathtub can be used)
" Water (stored regularly, away from the sunlight, and replaced every year if unused)
" Enough water for any pets

FIRE

You will need fire for warmth (covered above) and for cooking. Some off-grid options you can consider for cooking, and supplies, are:

¨ BBQ Grill (keep outdoors and remember to stock up on charcoal or propane)

¨ Camping Stoves

¨ Fireplace or Wood Burning Stove

¨ Natural Fuel Rocket Stoves

¨ Fuel for each selected option

¨ Metal cooking utensils

FOOD

Do not assume the grocery shelves will be stocked. Stock your own shelves with simple, sensible and smart emergency food choices, in advance. An important note on freezers: Avoid food poisoning. If the freezer temperature rises above 40 degrees for more than 2 hours, then throw away any perishable food. Also, keep track of expiration dates on al stockpiled food.

¨ Open and eat meals (little to no preparation, no refrigeration required, and with a long shelf life)

¨ Emergency food rations

¨ Reconstituted foods (remember some of them need boiling water)

¨ Freeze Dried/Dehydrated Meals (10+ years shelf life, such as Mountain House, Wise Foods, and Backpacker's Pantry)

¨ Military Meals Ready to Eat (MREs – high in calories, long shelf life, and easy to prepare)

¨ Store-Bought Canned Goods/Packaged Foods (easy to add to weekly grocery list, ready to eat, with many meat, vegetable and fruit options)

¨ Can opener and 2 backups

¨ Can Your Own Food (more complex, not recommended unless you're already a pro at it)

¨ Hunting, Farming food and animals, Gardening, and Gathering for food (more dicey in a bug in situation, unless you live outside the city in a low human traffic area)

¨ Mix & Match the above

¨ Foods for special dietary needs in the household (babies, diabetics, seniors, pets, people with allergies, etc.)

FIRST AID

You will need basic first aid, supplies (and skills) to respond for major injury and illnesses in the family, and the prescription medications that you and your family depend on to live. These supplies and medicines need to be monitored and rotated just like food. Consider these critical supplies:

¨ Comprehensive first aid kit

¨ Disaster preparedness medical kit

¨ Prescription medications

¨ First aid course taken by 2 family members

¨ First aid instruction book

¨ Contacts/spare eye-glasses/solution

SELF DEFENSE

See bugging out instructions to begin.

Also remember that in desperate times, good people get desperate, and criminals get brazen.

Self-defense when bugging in requires plans for home security upgrades, self and family defense, and the right tools.

Home Security Upgrades or 'MacGyver-Like Retrofits'

Solid metal or wood doors – no decorative glass.

Dead-bolt on every outside door.

Inside mounted door bar for added security.

"Beware of Dog" sign even if you just have a cat or goldfish. Criminals are looking for easy targets.

Graffiti spray paint to make the house look abandoned

Upgraded door hardware with deep-set 3" screws

Exterior motion lights (solar-powered) – front and back

'Defensive' rose bushes below each ground-level window.

Upgraded window locks / cut wood-block stoppers for inside.

Well-advertised video alarm system – whether you have one or not.

Family Self-Defense Tools & Training

¨ Guns (great for family defense; get some training with shotguns and handguns, then find the one you prefer and keep it in a locked box with the ammunition.)

¨ Knives

¨ Pepper spray

¨ Stun guns

HOME PRESERVATION ESSENTIALS WHEN BUGGING IN

1. Know how to turn off your utilities. Don't get your house blown up, flooded or burned to the ground. Get the proper tools (and knowledge) to quickly and safely disconnect all of your utilities.

2. Have a 'solution' when the garbage and sewage services go down. Store extra heavy-duty trash bags for human and pet waste, and for trash, just in case. Remember, hygiene and sanitation can save you or kill you. A 5-gallon bucket lined with a thick plastic garbage bag makes a suitable makeshift toilet.

IN CLOSING

It is truly my hope that by using these lists, you will be more prepared to protect yourself and your family from Ebola. If you do nothing else after reading this book, at least review the lists and see what you have already in your home. Stock up on what you can. Do what you can for your family. Be as prepared as you can.

Fail to plan, plan to die.

STAY CONNECTED TO GET MORE SURVIVAL LISTS

Thank you for reading through *Ebola Pandemic Survival Lists*!
Want to save time checking items off your lists?
Visit my Amazon aStore at http://astore.amazon.com/jakesalive-20 to see some of the fast and convenient options you have for buying your Ebola pandemic emergency supplies. It will also give you a good place to comparison shop, if you look for your items locally.
Want to be first in line to get other critical survival LISTS?
The next book in the series is: *Zombie Apocalypse Survival Lists*. Get Jake S. Alive updates on free eBooks and other new books right in your inbox, by signing up here:
http://forms.aweber.com/form/31/2065881531.htm